PELVIC FLOOR PHYSICAL THERAPY SERIES:
PREGNANCY BOOK 2

YOUR BEST BODY AFTER BABY

A POSTPARTUM GUIDE TO EXERCISE, SEX, AND PELVIC FLOOR RECOVERY

BY

JEN TORBORG, PT, DPT

First Edition: June 2018

ISBN-13: 978-1725926776
ISBN-10: 1725926776

Medical Disclaimer

None of the content in this book constitutes medical advice, nor is it a substitute for personalized health care. It is intended for informational and educational purposes only and is not to be construed as medical advice or instruction. If you have concerns about any medical condition, diagnosis, or treatment, you should consult with a licensed health care provider. If you are experiencing a medical emergency, you should call 911 immediately.

Jen Torborg assumes no responsibility or liability for any consequences resulting directly or indirectly from any action or inaction you take based on the information in or material linked to this book.

Pregnancy Red Flags

If something ever feels wrong, trust that feeling and talk to your health care provider right away, especially if you're experiencing any of the following:

*heavy vaginal bleeding that increases each day rather than decreases; large clots

*pain in legs with redness or swelling

*sore breasts that are red or feel hot to touch

*chills or fever

*changes to vision, severe headache, dizziness

*painful or difficulty with urination

*vaginal discharge with strong odor

*heart palpitations, difficulty breathing, chest pains

*have thoughts of harming yourself or your baby

THE LOTUS

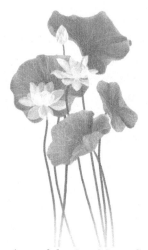

Artwork by Ana-Maria Cosma

The lotus grows out of the muddy waters into a beautiful flower. The opening of its leaves represent an expanding of the soul. This awakening symbolizes your growth and the ability to rise above obstacles. This plant was chosen to represent your precious and resilient time in the fourth trimester.

CONTENTS

INTRODUCTION

So you want your best body after baby? You want to understand what's going on with your body postpartum? You want to feel empowered in your healing?

I want that for you too!

There are quotes throughout this book from other pregnancy and postnatal professionals to complement the message I seek to bring you. Links to more information from these women are in the Resources appendix.

I want you to begin this book by soaking in these words of wisdom from Brianna Battles (she posted this one month postpartum) on body image and taking back your healing during this time:

> "I'm so proud of this body... look how incredible it is! In one month, I went from carrying a 10-pound baby in my belly to holding that baby in my arms as my organs reset, as my incision heals, as my diastasis begins rehab, as my breasts nourish, as my mind endures, as my rest decreases, as my heart grows with unconditional love for this baby boy. I trust the process my body is going through. I trust the time and patience it takes to recover and progress. I know how fast this goes. I know this time with a newborn is fragile, and my body can't be my focus, my obsession, my fear. I am not willing to let that mindset distract me from the little soul I get to care for and adjust to. My body will come back. My athleticism and routines will come back. My clothes will fit again. But this unique time in my life as a mother will never come back... and this time I'm doing everything I can to be in it, to enjoy it, treasure it. Because suddenly, that precious baby turns into a wild little boy. I see that reality daily! I know what's ahead!

Therefore, I refuse to let insecurities and obsession take away from honoring and respecting this chapter in my life and his. This baby deserves all of my obsession. And this mother deserves to embrace *all* chapters of her womanhood without aesthetics being the focus or concern."

—Brianna Battles, MS, CSCS

My goal is to help you achieve your best body after baby but in the most functional sense from a pelvic floor physical therapist (PT) perspective so that you feel better prepared and empowered to tackle your postpartum recovery. Many women don't even know what a pelvic floor PT is, yet in other countries postpartum rehab with a professional is the norm. In France, most new moms attend perineum rehabilitation within six weeks postpartum and are usually given ten to twenty visits. This can help new moms feel better physically and mentally and prevent problems further down the road by taking the time to heal now. Once a baby is born in the United States, most appointments are focused on the baby and not mom. Having a supportive team of professional caregivers, friends, and family near postpartum to help you is key. I hope this book will help you navigate this portion of your journey.

What is pelvic floor rehab postpartum? It is guiding a woman to improve her recovery of the pelvic floor and her whole body. Pelvic floor PT may include guiding you back to doing functional and exercise-related movements, enjoying sex pain free, helping you to stop from peeing your pants, and getting your bowel movements back on track.

I'm a physical therapist who specializes in pelvic floor PT. I have my Certificate of Achievement in Pelvic Health Physical Therapy (CAPP-Pelvic) and Certificate of Achievement in Pregnancy/Postpartum Physical Therapy (CAPP-OB) from the American Physical Therapy Association (APTA).

If you haven't already read my first book, *Your Best Pregnancy Ever*, I encourage you to do so. The book includes nine healthy habits to empower you such as embracing your breath, knowing your pelvic floor, and practicing self-care. These habits will be helpful postnatal as well. You completed a major life event, and your body will never be the same again, but that doesn't mean you shouldn't be able to gain back your strength, function, confidence, and happiness. Process letting go of what was and get excited about what is to come.

You now have new motivating factors such as your little one to drive you to be healthy and strong. But how do you plan to get there safely and intentionally?

I hope this book helps guide you through self-awareness and healing and that you're able to get more in tune with your vulva, pelvic floor, and your whole body. And that if something feels off, you'll feel more empowered to speak up.

> "I had to heal myself first: severe tearing in two places that led to an altered appearance of my vagina and vulva. Pain with intercourse that made penetration comfortable in only one position for over a year. Urine leakage with exercise. A three-finger width diastasis recti. Prolapse. This laundry list of dysfunction used to be the story of my body. It is not my story any longer. I went to a pelvic floor physical therapist, and it felt cold and overly medicalized. I felt vulnerable, like my body was a problem. I was shown how to do some Kegels, and I was told to return the next week. I cried during my session, and the therapist looked at me blankly and seemed uncomfortable. I left that office and didn't ever return. I knew healing in my body would not come in this environment, but at the time, I didn't know of any other paths. I became a pelvic floor physical therapist first and foremost so I could learn what I needed to learn to be able to heal myself. The healing I now offer others comes from a place of compassion and shared experience. With reverence and gratitude, I respectfully draw from traditions and thinkers outside of the medical model in addition to using some of the same techniques that worked to heal my own issues."
>
> —Dr. Jaime Goldman, DPT, RYT, Doula

Throughout the book, I often recommend having a pelvic floor PT or other professionals be part of your team during your recovery in healing and understanding your body. However, I want you to find someone you feel you work well with and connect with. You may feel limited in options based on your location or finances, but please always advocate for yourself. You deserve care from people who listen to you and respect you.

You got this, mama.

Best of luck in your fourth trimester healing!

This book does use cisnormative language. I am a white, heterosexual, able-bodied, cis woman and this is where I feel comfortable speaking from due to my own life experiences, although I do want to acknowledge that sex anatomy and gender are different. There is relevant information for all postpartum people in this book, but the subject matter and terminology is aimed at cis women.

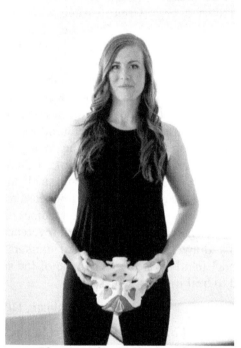

Photo credit: Kelsey Lindsey

CHAPTER 1:
REST AND HEALING

This chapter was by far the hardest for me to write because everyone's experience during childbirth is different. This may lead to your early days postpartum also being very different physically and emotionally. Everyone's personal life differs. Some moms have a great supportive team around them, some have difficulties in their family ties, and some may be on their own. For some moms, this is their first baby. Some have many kids already at home wanting their attention. Some moms are the financial breadwinner of their family and may feel pressured to get back at work right away. Some moms may not have to physically leave home to go to work but may have to care for others. I'm writing this book as someone who lives in the United States where we have no guaranteed paid maternity leave. So as much as I want this chapter to be about the ideal healing phase for you, I understand that this may not be possible for everyone. I'm sorry that not everyone can have access to this type of recovery. But I do want to highlight what healing in the early days and weeks postpartum could be like and why. If taking time to rest and heal can be part of your recovery, consider embracing this option.

The time after having a baby and getting back out there has many historical and cultural implications. Some cultures have specific practices for postpartum recovery: time for rest physically and mentally, support, limited or no entertaining, warmth, minimal movement, and healthy foods and fluids. Some women have been robbed of this time of healing over the years due to lack of support and community, slavery, expectations, lack of choice, etc. But if you have the freedom and ability to cultivate this precious time for healing, please do.

"In these early stages we want *lots of rest*. I don't want to get all preachy here, ladies, but you've *got* to rest in the early weeks wherever possible. Listen to your body and don't feel guilty about lying down and putting your feet up — literally! Pregnancy, labor (some will labor prior to having a cesarean), surgery, general anesthesia, sleep deprivation, feeding your baby, hormones... whoa, that is a *lot* for someone to go through. So please, please, please, give yourself the time and space to rest and heal. I find that women actually recover *faster* by starting out *slower*!"

—Marika Hart, PT, BSc, MSc

There's an old wives' tale: two weeks around the bed, two weeks around the house, two weeks around the community. I delved into research to see if there was any merit to this, as I often see a wide variety in how quickly or slowly new moms get back out there.

What I've gathered is that this time is extremely important for healing organs and tissues. You might not realize how much you need to heal. It is important that your body heals so that you have the strength and endurance you need to care for yourself and baby. Physically, the uterus expands roughly 15 times its normal size while you're pregnant. It will take four to six weeks for the uterus to contract back down to its normal size. At first, there is also a dinner plate-sized wound on the uterus from where the placenta was attached that needs to heal. There was pressure on your cervix, vagina, diaphragm, and abdominal muscles while you were pregnant. Regardless of the way you birthed (vaginal or cesarean), these tissues and muscles also need time to decrease in swelling to fully function again. This will also take about four to six weeks. You may also have encountered tears and/or stitches, which might require specific care and restrictions.

This is not a time to push through and get things done on your to-do list or entertain. And although I'm all about listening to your body, you might have some expectations for yourself that make you think you should do more than what you are ready for. As you start to feel better, try not to overdo things, which could set back your recovery.

So my advice is to listen to the old wives' tale in a way that fits your life. There is indeed some merit in its relation to your physical and mental healing. During your time around the bed, around the house, and around the community, I will give you some information about how to slowly prepare and transition your body into activity.

Throughout this whole time, it's important to attempt to get sleep, rest, fresh air, hydrate with water, and get plenty of nutrient-dense foods.

"I wish someone would have told me just how exhausted I would be the first few weeks of being home and caring for a new life. I was not prepared for how my brain would not be sharp, and simple tasks would be complicated simply due to the sleep deprivation. It sounds silly, but I actually made a list of good and healthy foods to eat when I was hungry so that I wouldn't have to remember or make decisions when it was time to eat. Check the list, check the refrigerator, eat. I also gave myself credit for simple tasks on a daily to-do list that included drinking at least 80 ounces of water, going outside, taking a shower. Being a task-oriented person, I found this helpful and calming for my brain."

—Meagan Peeters-Gebler, PT, DPT, CMTPT, CSCS

TWO WEEKS AROUND THE BED

During this time, it's important to rest and also to move in gentle ways. Moving your feet up and down (ankle pumps) can help increase circulation and decrease risk of blood clots. You could also elevate your feet to decrease swelling. Have others do household chores and bring the baby to you. Resist the temptation to do more. Just taking small walks to improve your mood and blood flow can be a gentle way to introduce movement and wake up your muscles. Take small resting breaks outdoors or with a window open for fresh air.

You may want to consider wrapping or binding for abdominal and/or pelvic floor support. There are a lot of different methods out there including belly wraps and high-waisted compression shorts. These can be helpful for healing and support, but if the wrap is too tight, it could exacerbate pressure on a healing pelvic floor. Consider working with a PT or your provider to decide if it's a helpful choice for you and if it's being fit correctly. Either way, it's more important to start waking up your own stability system with gentle voluntary muscle contractions.

To do this, focus on diaphragm breathing and getting to know your pelvic floor muscles again. (Lots of this in book one and more in the next chapter.) You can do this in isolated positions such as lying down, sitting, or standing. You can also begin to add it in with your functional movements, such as sitting up in bed, lifting your baby, and standing up from the chair. Use a log roll to get up slowly from the bed. Sit down on the side of your bed, and gently swing your legs up to the bed together in a bent position while you lower your upper half to the bed. This should result in you lying on your side. Do the reverse movement to get out of bed. This can help decrease pressure on your expanding belly and back.

"Learning to coordinate my breath with my daily movements was the most beneficial piece of information I received regarding my body after baby. After our first child, I hurt my back, which bothered me for years, and after our second child, I split my recti muscles, both because I was not lifting and moving appropriately. Once I began using my breath with my movements, I stopped having trouble with both. I now naturally use my exhales during exertion, which is so much easier on my body and also very empowering! I feel powerful when I use my breath, I can actually accomplish more tasks, and I was able to strengthen my pelvic floor, which in turn made me feel strong and confident in my ability to strengthen the rest of my body too."

—Malari, Certified Educator of Infant Massage

Prioritize these tips from the first book:

1. **Sleep**. Attempt to sleep when your baby does. Ask someone to watch the baby or help bring the baby to you for feedings so that you can sleep when possible. Try to use time where your baby is sleeping to catch up on rest rather than the dishes. Your physical and mental health will thank you.

2. **Hydrate**. Drink plenty of water especially while breastfeeding. Water, water, water. It's free if you live in an area where you have access to clean tap or well water. If your water isn't clean (check with a testing kit), then consider buying a filtration system so that you have unlimited access to water. Get a reusable water bottle. Put your water bottle where you usually nurse. Drink up. Hydration will help with your healing and bowel movements!

3. **Eat nutrient-dense food**. Eat vegetables, fruits, nuts, seeds, healthy fats, and proteins. Eat foods that give you energy and nourish you. Eating nutritious foods will help you heal.

4. **Advocate for yourself.** Have emotional support available to you personally and professionally if needed. Know that if something doesn't feel quite right mentally or emotionally, you're best to talk it through with someone so that you're not alone and have resources to help you through this transition in your life.

Pain relief measures

Ice for the first 48 hours. Consider soaking a maxi pad in water and witch hazel, then freeze for a healing frozen maxi pad. After the first two days, switch to sitz baths. A sitz bath is when you fill a tub or basin with tepid water and sit in it for up to twenty minutes a few times a day. This can clean the perineum area (the area between your vulva and anus), decrease swelling, and help to relieve pain. Consider adding ½ cup Epsom salt and ½ cup sea salt to the sitz bath to improve healing of the tissues. You may want to add essential oils to the sitz bath as well.

"Using a squirt bottle or peri bottle to prerinse your perineal area prior to urination can be really helpful in minimizing any burning or stinging you may feel after a perineal tear. Avoid wiping the area initially and pat dry instead."

—Kelly Diehl, PT, DPT

Get your bowels moving

Your first poop will not be as bad as you might think it will be. The longer you wait, though, the harder it will get, so when you start to feel an urge to poop, listen to it. It can help to use a pillow to provide compression on your abdominal muscles to assist them in regulating the pressure of this region, especially if you're healing from a cesarean incision. Improve your bowel movements with drinking lots of water, eating plenty of fiber, and taking calcium and magnesium supplements.

"Calcium and magnesium supplements (which women should take in pregnancy and postpartum — really, all Westerners should take [them] because our diet is so lacking in them) is a natural stool softener, thus a great alternative to over-the-counter softeners that mess up your body and gut. The magnesium also helps with postpartum cramping."

—Chelsea Fanchi, doula

Use a Squatty Potty or some sort of stool to put your feet up on so that your knees are higher than your hips. You can also work on stretching your muscles near your pelvis, low back, and abdomen. Work on deep breathing to massage your colon from the inside. Deep breathing or diaphragm breathing consists of taking full, symmetrical breaths that fill your chest, belly, ribs to the sides, and ribs to the back equally and calmly, then slowly letting the air out on an exhale. Take some small walks to loosen things up. You could massage your abdomen and low back.

When you're ready to have your bowel movement, remember to breathe. Don't strain, push, or hold your breath. Breathe out as you gently bear down and relax, and lengthen your pelvic floor muscles. Sometimes splinting your perineum, which means putting pressure on the area between your vaginal opening and anus, can be helpful. This can provide comfort and support while reestablishing body awareness and easing apprehension with lengthening your pelvic floor.

And if that's not working, you could always try stool softeners or laxatives. It's important to get those bowels moving. Without consistent bowel movements, you can build up pressure inside your body, which can potentially contribute to back pain, hip/pelvic pain, pelvic organ prolapse, and urinary leakage.

Two Weeks Around The Home

"How do you return to exercise after childbirth? First you breathe, then you walk. After the first few weeks of initial postpartum recovery and starting diaphragmatic breathing, the next step is to start moving to promote circulation to your pelvic floor and abs, to aid digestion and constipation, to strengthen your hips and legs, and to lift your mood and get you out of your home. Start around two weeks postpartum and take it slow. I see women who are getting their body back two weeks after childbirth. There is no medal for who recovers fastest from childbirth. It's hard work to slow down, but we have to respect the process of recovery. It is a marathon, not a sprint. So take it slow and be kind to yourself. Your vagina will thank you."

—Sara Reardon, PT, DPT, WCS, BCB-PMD

Start to slowly increase the frequency of walks or the length of walks you are taking. Start to take back some of your typical household chores mindfully. Take breaks when you need them or before you truly need them. Think of your posture, breath, and pelvic floor while performing these tasks. Think about how much effort these tasks will take if you can break it down into a few steps or take some breaks before doing the whole chore at once.

TWO WEEKS AROUND THE COMMUNITY

Begin reading the chapter on returning to exercise for how you can approach further movement. Start to check out the chapter on scar tissue as it heals. Begin getting out of the house a bit more but in small, manageable time frames. Start small and build up gradually rather than feeling like you've pushed it too far. Remember to make time for sleep, hydration, and nutritious foods. Continue to ask for help from others.

Recap:

1. Resting in the early days and weeks is important for the actual physical and mental healing process.

2. You can improve your healing by sleeping, hydrating, eating nutritious foods, using pain relief ideas for your perineum, having regular bowel movements, and easing back into activity.

3. Start with simple exercises like diaphragm breathing, gentle pelvic floor exercises, and walking. (More on that in the next chapter.)

CHAPTER 2:
RETURNING TO EXERCISE

Everyone's journey back to exercise will be different physically and mentally. Show yourself and other moms grace during this period. Each new mom will heal at different rates, and although it's important for your body to heal the first few weeks, no judgment should be cast on one another for how quickly or slowly one returns to fitness. Hopefully, the education in the previous chapter highlights the importance of why it's key to be intentional in your healing postpartum. And then it's up to you to know your own body and mind and what your limitations and modifications will be. Ask for help if you're not sure.

Your return to exercise will vary greatly based upon

- your previous exercise level

- any complications during pregnancy, labor, and birth (including tearing, stitches, cesarean, intensity of labor, trauma)

- how well your pelvic floor and abdominal muscles are healing or working

- mental state: some may experience a tough time holding themselves back from pushing too hard, and others may have a hard time motivating themselves to get moving in a meaningful way

Whatever your fitness goals may be now, it's important to have a plan. If you've ever watched someone recover from a major trauma, surgery, or bed rest, there's often a guided rehab protocol that one would move through slowly and steadily. As your initial exercises get easier, then continue to advance them. Being postpartum, you have a new normal, and therefore it's great to have an actual game plan. Maybe even write it out. I'll go through a few examples of returning to cardio and strength training. Modify the suggestions to fit your interests and level of fitness.

In the first book *Your Best Pregnancy Ever*, there is a chapter that details what's normal versus common and what to look for while listening to your body. There should be no pain, no leakage, and no feelings of pelvic heaviness or falling out. You also should not see any doming, coning, or bulging along the linea alba, the vertical midline of your abdomen between the six-pack abs. If any of the functional activities (sit to stand, lifting, bending) or exercises (jumping, running, strength training) you participate in cause these common but not normal symptoms, consider backing off and finding a modification. You want to be able to move intentionally without causing the symptoms. Ask for help if you need it.

"This means we have to slow down and be a little more mindful about how we move, but I promise you it's worth it and your vagina will thank you."

—Sara Reardon, PT, DPT, WCS, BCB-PMD

Let's begin

If you haven't already, begin to connect with your diaphragm breathing, posture, and pelvic floor muscles to set yourself up for success during your exercises. There are detailed chapters on breath, posture, and the pelvic floor in the first book. But here's a recap of what to work on fitnesswise, even in your first days postpartum.

Connect with your breath

Your diaphragm, the breathing muscle along the bottom of the ribs and the muscle that represents the roof of the core, most likely became tightened and constricted while your baby was growing. Now is your chance to make sure you can find a nice, full breath again. Take a breath in, and you should feel not only your chest and belly expand, but also your ribs to the sides and in the back. When you exhale and let the air out, those areas should sink back down. Inhale = expand in all directions; exhale = relax, sink back down.

As you move your body from a sitting position to standing, while you lift your baby, or while you reach for something, practice exhaling (blowing the air out of your mouth) during the exertion.

Take a full breath in and then exhale and move. This is an easy way to optimize the pressure inside your body and start getting your core muscles, pelvic floor, and lower abdomen to coordinate again. Some cues that might help you remember to do this without making it a forceful exhalation and to avoid gripping your abdominals would be to pretend you are cooling soup on a spoon or blowing out through a straw when you move.

Posture

Your posture may have changed while you were pregnant to accommodate your growing baby, but now that baby is out and being carried around, you may notice that you still fall back into pregnancy posture. Changing up your posture itself is an exercise. Try to find a relatively neutral pelvic position most of the time, meaning you don't want to tuck your tailbone/butt under and have a flat back, but you also don't want to untuck to the extreme and arch your back to the max. Go between those two directions a few times, and then try to find the middle ground. Most new moms tend to live with their butt tucked under, so try to untuck and use those glutes (your butt muscles)! Now that your pelvis can move more easily, try to align your ribs over your pelvis. This will optimize your body's pressure system inside the core (diaphragm on top, pelvic floor on the bottom). Ribs over the pelvis means not leaning so far back that your ribs are flared forward and not so rounded forward in your chest and shoulders that there's no room in the core.

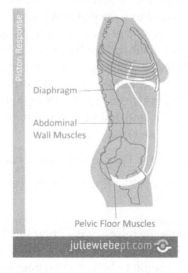

Piston Response

Diaphragm

Abdominal Wall Muscles

Pelvic Floor Muscles

juliewiebept.com

The concept of a pressure relationship between the diaphragm and the pelvic floor (and much more!) is taught as Piston Science created and owned by Julie Wiebe, PT. For over 20 years, she has been integrating these concepts and strategies into movement, function, and all forms of fitness, including running, CrossFit and more. Julie has also been an advocate for empowering women to pursue fitness in the midst of pelvic health and pain issues. She is internationally recognized for pioneering the integrative approach that is now widely relied upon by physical therapists and fitness professionals, including me. Her information is used with permission. For more information about Julie, please visit her website, blogs, videos, and online courses. Links are located in the Resources appendix.

Pelvic floor

Your pelvic floor muscles are those that connect from the pubic bone in the front to the tailbone in the back and your sit bones side to side. They are internal muscles that wrap around all three openings (urethra, vagina, anus) and attach to various depths in that region. It is a group of muscles that work together to keep your organs up and inside of you, to keep you from leaking, and to provide support and stability.

To begin connecting with your pelvic floor, find the diaphragm breath we just talked about, and add a relaxation of the pelvic floor with your inhale and a contraction of the pelvic floor with your exhale. It's also important to sometimes practice lengthening your pelvic floor on an exhale to help you relax when urinating or having a bowel movement. To focus on the relax portion, visualize your pelvic floor letting go, melting like butter, opening like a flower. To focus on the contraction portion, visualize yourself closing your vaginal opening around a kidney bean and lifting the bean up and into your body, stopping from peeing, stopping from passing gas, pulling the pubic bone and tailbone up and into your body, and pulling the sit bones up and into your body.

- Inhale = relax pelvic floor = let kidney bean go.
- Exhale = contract pelvic floor = lift the kidney bean up and in.
- Repeat.

Start these pelvic floor exercises in isolation the first few days while you're resting your body. Try them while feeding your baby, while in the shower, or before going to bed. As you connect with the area and start to feel stronger, start to add the concept to movements: getting up from the chair, lifting your baby, and bending down to pick something up from the floor.

Over time, you will want the ability to contract, relax, and lengthen your pelvic floor in all types of positions and movements. You'll want to be able to contract not only on an exhale but also with an inhale. You'll learn to be able to do quick contractions of your pelvic floor muscles faster than a breath and endurance contractions more than 10 seconds (longer than a typical exhale). All the different ways you can work your pelvic floor muscles are in my first book in the chapter "Know Your Pelvic Floor." Remember, pelvic floor contractions (doing a Kegel) does not mean tightening your butt cheeks, squeezing your thighs together, holding your breath, or squeezing your upper abs or bearing down. To get your strength back, you should avoid constant clenching of your abdominals and pelvic floor. It's so important that this area, like all other muscles, can find a balance between activation and relaxation. If you aren't sure if you are performing pelvic floor exercises correctly, seek out feedback from a professional such as a pelvic floor PT.

Putting it together

As we start to plan out our return to exercise, please keep this strategy in mind. In any exercise you try — walking, lifting, running, rowing, jumping — you should be able to feel yourself find a full breath and that your pelvic floor can follow your breath and contract and relax as you need it to.

Add this strategy to simple movements with only five to ten repetitions with a focus on quality.

The strategy of inhale + relax, then exhale + contract + move can be applied to following real life activities, as exercises, before you begin your full return to exercise:

1. Sit to stand from a chair

2. Lifting baby

3. Picking up an object from the ground

4. Lifting your car seat or stroller in and out of the car

"Movement is important, but listen to your body and be patient with yourself. Ligaments can remain somewhat lax throughout breastfeeding, which can contribute to feelings of pelvic pressure or heaviness in early postpartum. This may be more problematic after activity or intercourse. Learning to reconnect with your core and being aware of body mechanics during activity can help reduce some of these feelings. After my son was born, I would even use gravity to combat pelvic pressure after overactivity. I would lay him on the floor to play and position myself on forearms and knees with my hips in the air. The beautiful thing about pelvic floor contractions is that you do them while playing with your kiddo(s). This helped me connect with my core and reduce the pressure I felt through my pelvis."

—Kelly Diehl, PT, DPT

RETURN TO CARDIO

The ways you can vary your progression include: distance, total time, speed, and predictable versus variable terrain/conditions.

Example for returning to walking, jogging, running, hiking

1. Start with small frequent walks: five minutes in length at a slow to normal speed. After a few days like this with no feelings of pain, leakage or falling out, start to increase time or distance.

2. Progress walks to be ten to fifteen minutes at your normal speed.

3. Continue to lengthen the time of your walks in five- to ten-minute increments at your normal speed.

4. Advance the total time of your walks or start to vary speed in intervals. If your end goal is jogging or running, you can start to add in very small intervals of jogging a block or 30 seconds to a minute, then return to walking for a few minutes before once again jogging for a short period of time. You should continue checking in with your body during and after these advancements to monitor for pain, leakage, or pelvic heaviness.

5. Continue to change up lengthening the speed portions of jog/run with walking to slowly build up to more jogging/running than walking.

6. Vary terrain to trails, hills, and uneven surfaces as you feel stronger.

The example above could take some new moms weeks or months or years. It really depends so much on how your body is responding. This is different from one woman to the next and from one pregnancy to the next. Leaking or feeling like something is falling out is not something to push through. You may find that you can increase your time just fine, but once you add in speed, you start to leak. Or maybe it's not the change of speed, but at a certain distance or on hills you notice symptoms. Stop and modify. Keep staying active, but don't push into the symptoms. If they aren't resolving on their own or with your intentional pelvic floor exercises, breath, and posture, reach out to a professional specializing in postpartum recovery (links in Resources appendix) to get an assessment and develop a plan specific to your needs.

RETURN TO STRENGTH

The ways you can vary your progression include: weights, body position, repetitions, sets, total time, and intensity or speed.

Example for squats

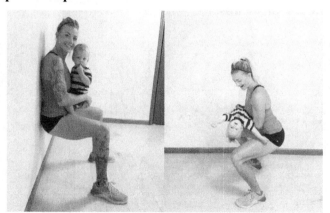

1. Start with holding on to a countertop, railing, sturdy chair, or with your back against a wall. Work on getting your form, breath, and pelvic floor coordinated with the movement. Perform a maximum of ten repetitions at one time so you can focus on quality. Slowly increase repetitions by five or by the number of times you're performing the squats per day.

2. Advance by performing squats without weight yet, but no holding on anymore. Perform to a depth you feel comfortable with and continue to focus on form, breath, and pelvic floor.

Continue to perform only ten repetitions. Increase repetitions over time by five or by number of times you're performing per day.

3. Start to add weights to your squats. Hold your baby or pick something less than 20 pounds to start with. Perform squats with the weight or baby around chest height. Continue to add reps/sets as it gets easier. Continue to have a strong focus on quality and no pain, leakage, or feelings of falling out.

4. If that's your goal, continue to increase weights — barbell, kettlebell, water jugs, baby, etc. — in different positions, keeping the weight light and getting used to different lifts again. Ensure quality and connection to the pelvic floor with no symptoms.

5. Ease back into whatever your new squat goals are — depth, reps, weight, speed, etc. Continue to listen to your body. Vary challenges by performing single leg squats or adding a rotational component.

Again, the example above may take some women weeks, months, or years to progress through, based on their own unique circumstances.

Example for push-ups

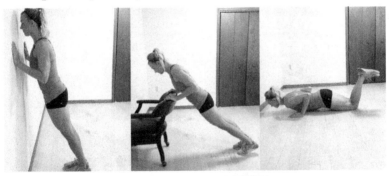

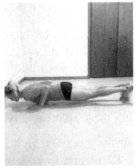

1. Start doing push-ups against a wall or countertop and focus on breath and pelvic floor coordination.

2. Continue to increase repetitions at the previous height or decrease distance to floor.

3. Progress to floor push-ups from knees or plank position. Keep reps low at five to ten as you focus on form, breath, and pelvic floor.

4. Continue to increase total reps/sets or challenge yourself with different placements of your hands.

Example for plank progression

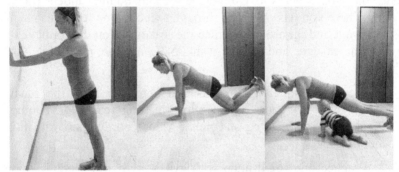

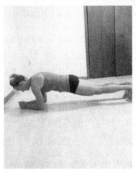

1. Start in a modified position similar to push-up positions: on the wall, countertop, or couch if needed. Time the length of your plank with just one or two breath cycles to begin rather than counting total time in the plank position. Breath cycle: inhale and exhale gently (don't hold your breath).

2. Increase the number of breath cycles in those positions, and then slowly make your way to the floor. Plank from knees. Plank using straight arms. Plank using forearms. Monitor for symptoms

and doming/coning of the abdomen, and continue to connect with pelvic floor, breath, and posture.

3. As you're able to hold the plank position longer, add in more functional challenges. You could add movement of arms with shoulder taps, reaching out, or alternate between forearm and hands during the hold. Or you could add movement of the legs with leg lifts up or tap a leg to the side.

Return to jumping

Just because you had a baby does not mean you're doomed to exile from the trampoline for fear of peeing your pants, nor does it mean that you should perform jumping jacks and double unders (jump roping where you pass the rope through twice in one jump) as much as you want and ignore or embrace the leakage. You do not have to live with leakage, and if you want to be able to jump dry, you should!

1. Start with squatting, and as you come up from the squat, extend up onto your toes to mimic getting ready for a jump. Practice your breathing and pelvic floor coordination with this modification.

2. Practice one small jump with exhale and with a pelvic floor contraction during the takeoff and landing.

3. Slowly increase the height of the jump *or* the number of jumps in a row. For example, breathe in, then exhale/jump twice, then inhale-relax-break, then exhale/jump twice, then rest. Slowly increase the number of jumps in a row or height of the jump very intentionally so that you can notice specifically where/if you have any symptoms occur. Is it just on higher jumps, is it the takeoff versus the landing, or is it just past rep eight?

If you know when symptoms are occurring, you'll be able to better modify and not push past the limitations of what your body is capable of. If you're having trouble getting back into this, work with a pelvic floor PT or postnatal fitness specialist, who can help you with a more thorough assessment of what you have going on and the coordination and timing.

Hopefully, you're able to use the above progressions to modify the exercises you enjoy doing and come up with a plan of how to ease back into your movements intentionally. If you are experiencing any pain, leakage, pelvic heaviness, or coning/doming, reach out for help. It does not necessarily mean your muscles are weak! There's a lot at play including your connective tissues' role in healing. Difficulty with the coordination may include: ability to contract and relax your pelvic floor and abdominal muscles, tight muscles or scar tissue, and injury/trauma sustained during labor/birth. Lots of times you'll be able to play detective and modify your program yourself, but don't be scared or worried if you run into some of these. There's help out there to get you back on track physically and mentally with your exercise goals!

And keep exercise fun. You should enjoy moving in ways that make you feel strong and healthy. I love the following quote from Haley Shevener about getting in workouts at the playground. The link to her full blog post on this topic is in the Resources appendix.

"Many people who train with the intention of improving their general health and fitness will never need a simple piece of gym equipment. I work with clients in their homes, and sometimes I never even need to bring a single weight! We can use tables, chairs, jugs of water, and anything else that can be lifted, stood on, or moved. The one thing that can be challenging with home workouts is working on your upper-body pulling strength. The playground makes training pulling motions accessible and much simpler than dangling yourself off a dining room table (although I've been there too!). Bars, swings, ropes, and poles transform into places to do rows, flies, and pull-up movements. Equipment is usually placed at various heights, making the possibilities endless! Having a go at the monkey bars is pretty humbling if you haven't tried them since elementary school, but you can work up to all of these movements by changing the position of your body relative to the piece of equipment. Sometimes I talk to women who really want to start getting in more movement while at the playground but are afraid of the reactions they'll get from other parkgoers. I totally get it; it can feel like everyone is staring at you, unsure of why you're doing split squats on a park bench. If you want to get in some playground push-ups and planks, think of this as a great opportunity to work on building *your* confidence and practice doing *your* thing without worrying about what other people will think of you! It takes practice, but eventually, it will come naturally to you, and you'll probably find that other people don't care or are supportive of you (and that their opinion isn't the one that matters, either!)"

—Haley Shevener, CSCS

Recap:

1. Connect with your breath, posture, and pelvic floor. Return to exercise is about strategy, not necessarily the specific exercises you're performing.

2. Add in your breath and pelvic floor to daily functional movements: sit to stand, lifting, bending.

3. Plan to slowly ease back into your cardio goals. Consider writing out a plan.

4. Intentionally ease back into your strength training goals.

5. Continue to achieve everything you wish to as it pertains to exercise and fitness, keeping in mind quality and reaching out for help if you experience any pain, leakage, pelvic heaviness, or DRA coning/doming/bulging.

CHAPTER 3:
RETURNING TO SEX

Sex will probably feel different. And at first, depending on hormones and healing, there may be some slight discomfort that requires generous lubrication and easing into intercourse with strategy, but sex should not hurt. Painful sex is never normal at any point in life. Don't settle for the advice that you should drink some wine, take a bath, and try to relax a little. Don't settle for the advice that you should just push through and it will get better with time. There may be multiple physical and emotional components at play here.

- **Physical elements**: scar tissue, healing of muscles/tissue, hormones, tight muscles

- **Nervous system and emotional components**: guarding of the body from trauma experienced during labor and birth, guarding against the previous time you've tried sex that became painful, and getting comfortable with your new body

If your body perceives that something will be painful, regardless of whether there is actual tissue damage, it will most likely be painful. This chapter will cover advice on how you can get comfortable with your vulva and vagina yourself and with your partner. Just like with returning to exercise, the progression you move through will be based on listening to your own body and what it's ready for. Consider seeking out help with a pelvic floor PT, postnatal specialists, and mental health/sex therapists to deal with the various components of your recovery. Also, consider lube!

Your vulva and vagina are most likely drier than they were before due to hormones, especially if you are breastfeeding. There are a lot of lubricant options out there, but my advice is to read the labels. Some lubricants that are well marketed can actually dry you out more or may have irritating additives and fragrances. Look for options without glycerin or parabens, no flavors, fragrances, or tingling effects. Opt for water-based or silicone-based lubricants (Slippery Stuff, Good Clean Love, Yes!, Sliquid Organics, Uber Lube). Or consider coconut or olive oil from your kitchen cabinet, but remember oil doesn't mix well with condoms.

"If pregnancy and childbirth weren't enough to put your pelvic floor through the wringer, breastfeeding is another event that affects your vagina. To keep your breast milk supply up, your estrogen levels remain low. And low estrogen is pretty much like your vagina is in menopause, which is why your vagina feels like a desert during sex and your period doesn't return until breastfeeding decreases. Low estrogen means your vaginal tissues are dry, thin, and not as supportive until your estrogen levels increase as your baby gets older and requires less and less breastmilk. Pelvic floor PT can also help improve circulation to your pelvic floor, offer tips for vaginal dryness, and help your muscles stay strong to prevent leakage and prolapse, as your vagina is still in recovery phase while breastfeeding. So mommas, be patient, be kind to your vagina, and be proactive in its strengthening and healing phase by working with a pelvic floor PT during postpartum recovery."

—Sara Reardon, PT, DPT, WCS, BCB-PMD

Here are some examples of how you can ease back into intimacy with your partner. Choose ways that feel comfortable and appropriate for your goals. Often, our lack of awareness, comfort, and confidence in knowing this part of our body may contribute to fear, pain, and tension we feel.

Feeling yourself

1. Next time you're in the shower or have some time to lie down in a relaxed position, start by feeling your abdominal and pelvic region. Simply begin with the goal of feeling the tissues and muscles on the outside. If you had a cesarean birth, start to feel your lower abdomen and work on making peace with touching this area. For some this may be easy. For others, it's extremely triggering. The next chapter will cover scar tissue in more detail. If you're not ready to touch your scars yet, skip this part. Feel

around the rest of your belly. Feel the skin, the muscles, the stretch marks. Get comfortable with your own hands touching your body. Move on to your pelvic area. Touch your vulva. Feel the labia majora and the labia minora and the clitoris. Feel your way around externally and see if there are any painful areas. If so, work on gentle touching that area in a way that does not cause pain. Use gentle touch in a slow, intentional way to increase your positive experience in self-exploration rather than pushing through pain.

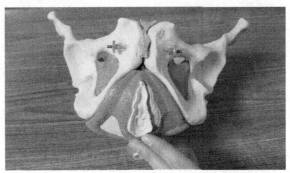

2. Progress by starting to feel internally. Do so gently. Pretend your vaginal opening is a clock with 12:00 being up towards the urethra/clitoris and 6:00 being towards the anus. Begin by slowly inserting one finger into your vagina towards the 6:00 position. Hold there for a bit and simply sense how it feels. Slowly move your finger towards the 3:00 position, then back to the 6:00, and then toward the 9:00 position. Take your time and try to make this a positive or at least neutral experience. Do not push into pain. Take full breaths as you're doing this and think positive thoughts.

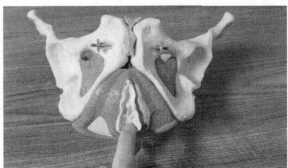

3. Advance to feel deeper and/or with more speed. Continue to feel in different directions and depths of your vagina. Use different pressures. Feel your pelvic floor muscles internally: contract, relax, and lengthen. Feel your breath gently expand and contract these muscles at a low level naturally. Notice if there are any areas that feel tight or painful and slowly work to bring gentle touch and release to those areas.

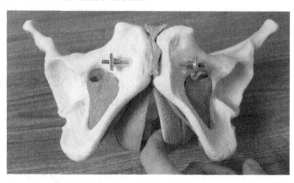

Continue to touch and feel internally and externally in any ways that you may encounter during sexual intercourse. Use this time to make peace with your body and experience physically and mentally. Note if there are certain areas that you will want to be careful and mindful of while returning to intercourse with your partner. Only pursue this exercise as a positive, pain-free experience. Other ways some women find helpful to advance at this point is using a dilator, wand, or sex toys at this point as progression to partner intimacy. Vibration has been shown to help with healing tissue and scars.

Sex and other forms of intimacy

When you feel ready and want to begin being intimate with your partner, have an open conversation about going slowly and speaking up if something doesn't feel right. You may not jump right back into positions or speeds you were used to previously. There may be different positions that are less painful and allow for you to feel more in control of the depth of penetration. There are lots of options as you heal physically and emotionally. As hormones settle back down and you work through the above steps, you should be able to return to sex pain free.

The same way you've worked through touching yourself slowly and intentionally may be something you want to work through with your partner. You may choose to start with external stimulation rather than any forms of penetration if that feels right for you. The more open and honest you can be, your partner can help you into making this a positive, pain-free activity you'll continue to enjoy in the long run. Don't put pressure on yourself to orgasm right away. Find ways to reach the orgasm externally with the clitoris rather than pushing through anything (friction, speed, positions, length of time) you're not ready for it internally.

Again, you should not push through pain. There are specific ways a pelvic floor PT can help you postpartum to work through the physical things at play. A PT can help you better understand how the nervous system and brain is responding in a protective way and how to work through that. Considering talking with a medical provider about hormone contribution if these methods are not helping dryness.

Every woman will get back to sex at different rates based on healing, hormones, and sex drive. Give yourself time and grace to connect with your pelvic floor muscles, breath, vulva, vagina, clitoris, and abdomen. You are beautiful and resilient. You've got this!

If you want more understanding on libido and desire, consider checking out these two great books: *Come As You Are* by Emily Nagoski and *Reclaiming Desire* by Andrew Goldstein, MD and Marianne Brandon, PhD.

Recap:

1. Start with feeling yourself gently externally and then internally to notice anything that feels off or painful. Try to create positive touch experiences.

2. Have an open and honest conversation with your partner about easing back into intercourse or other forms of intimacy.

3. Modify intimacy to find ways that are not painful as your body heals physically and mentally.

4. Reach out to a pelvic floor PT near you for an individualized assessment and treatment plan to get you back to pain-free intercourse!

CHAPTER 4:
OPTIMIZING SCAR TISSUE

There are a few different ways you may encounter scar tissue postpartum: in the perineum (the area between your vagina and anus), other parts of the vulva including the opening of the vagina (introitus), and the labia minora. Scars in this area may be from tearing during childbirth or an episiotomy. You may have some stitches depending on severity. Another area new moms may encounter scar tissue is from a cesarean birth in which layers of tissue in the lower abdomen including muscles were cut open to the uterus to birth the baby.

Scar tissue is what we call the connective tissue in areas that were damaged from injury or surgery. The tissue is laid down by the body during the healing process quickly in order to decrease exposure to outer elements and decrease chance of infection. This tissue has slightly different texture and mobility than an area of your body without a scar. The tissue changes as it repairs the area.

Sometimes as the tissue is repairing, it adheres to other tissue around it and can cause restrictions in mobility. We call these scar tissue adhesions, and these restrictions can sometimes contribute to pain or a decrease in your range of motion and strength in that area. The area of scars may also have some changes in sensitivity. You may notice pain, burning, tingling, or numbness. These things can all be worked on to improve the way your body feels and moves.

Your goal is to get the tissue in areas of scarring to move as freely as possible like other skin and tissue. You want that area to be pain free and to not be numb. You want to have a return of strength to that region so that your scars are not interfering with your function.

Sensitivity issues with scar tissue may be more than just physical in nature. It also may be your nervous system's response to the trauma you experienced during the injury or surgery. Your brain may have a heightened protective response to that area, so that even though you just barely touch an area of a scar, you feel increased pain that seems out of proportion to the touch your body felt. Some of this heightened response could be due to the emotions surrounding the cause of the scar. Was it an emergency cesarean birth that you are struggling to come to terms with? Was it an episiotomy that you so hoped to avoid?

There are many layers of healing involved here, and my advice is to go at a pace that feels comfortable to you. You do not need to rush into this portion of healing if you don't feel ready yet. Maybe you're ready to tackle the physical aspect but not the emotional trauma. Maybe you'd like to first work on the emotional trauma on your own or with a professional before starting to approach the physical aspects of scars.

The sooner you can work on the physical aspects of a scar, the easier it is to change the tissues. However, be open and honest with yourself and your provider about what you feel comfortable with. Some of scar tissue work may tap into discomfort briefly, but it should never be so painful that you're cringing or holding your breath. Aim for not letting pain increase above a 3 to 5 out of 10 (0 being no pain and 10 being the worst pain).

The physical restrictions for scar tissue may impede your body's ability to fully use the muscles around the area. This could potentially lead to pelvic floor dysfunction, painful intercourse, leakage, back pain, hip pain, or abdominal pain. It's important that eventually you feel like you can touch and move the areas of the scar without pain or disruption of function.

Below are examples of how to start working through the various scars physically and how to calm your nervous system. Find what works for you. And if you need it, reach out to a pelvic floor PT, postnatal massage therapist, or mental health counselor/therapist for more guided support.

Wait to start working on scar tissue until the scar has completely closed and you've been given the okay to begin by your provider. Typically, this is about a six-week wait for the healing to take place, sometimes sooner or longer depending on the severity of the scar and its ability to heal.

PERINEUM AND VULVA SCARS

1. Start by touching the scar externally at a pressure that does not bring on pain. For some, this might be going straight to touching the scar with their hands on the scar itself. For others, this may mean starting to touch above underwear or with a cotton ball for a lighter touch. Slowly work on increasing the time you feel comfortable touching the area and the amount of pressure.

2. Once the area feels okay with the touch of your fingers, start to press down on the scar and move it in different directions: up and down, side to side, clockwise and counterclockwise. Do this at different depths of the scar tissue and along different parts of the scar tissue.

3. Depending on where and how deep your scar goes, insert one finger inside the vagina to feel the scar internally and work the tissue inside and outside between your fingers. Roll the tissue between the fingers gently.

4. Continue to perform depths and directions you feel comfortable with for about five minutes every day until you no longer feel discomfort, numbness, or restrictions in the area.

CESAREAN SCARS

1. Start with gentle touch on top of the cesarean scar — this could initially be above clothing — or on skin using a Kleenex, cotton ball, or scarf to slowly touch along the scar. Begin to desensitize the area to general touch.

2. As the area is desensitized to general touch, you can begin to press down directly on the scar itself with your fingers at different depths. Start to press the tissue up and down, side to side, clockwise, and counterclockwise. Press the tissue above and below the scar in toward each other.

3. As the above movements start to feel easy and not restricted, move to slightly more aggressive techniques such as plucking. Plucking is picking up the scar in between your fingers and rolling the tissue together in a pinch. You can also add in skin

rolling where you pinch the skin between your index fingers and thumb with one or both hands, and then gently roll the skin with your index and middle fingers while your thumbs follow, keeping the skin pinched up.

4. Continue performing various scar massage and mobilization techniques daily for five minutes until you no longer feel pain, numbness, or restrictions in the area.

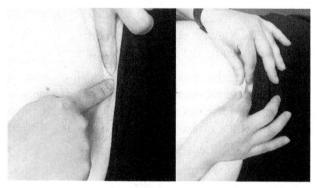

"Since about six weeks postpartum, I have been doing scar mobilization to try to help tolerate clothing. I just get in a comfy reclined position, drop a few drops of a blend of oils (frankincense, lavender, myrrh, rose in avocado carrier oil), and work on it for ten or so minutes."

—Abigail Inman, PT, DPT

Other things that may help with scars:

- dry needling by a physical therapist or chiropractor
- vitamin E oil and/or wheat germ oil
- kinesio tape or rock tape
- nutrition and supplements to support collagen and healing
- vibration

Recap:

1. Scar tissue may contribute to pain, numbness, and restrictions in movement and strength.

2. Working through the physical and emotional parts of scars will be helpful to your postpartum recovery.

3. Follow a gentle progression of working on scars with your hands or with a professional once the scar has healed.

CHAPTER 5:
LET'S TALK DIASTASIS RECTI

Diastasis recti abdominus (DRA) or diastasis recti is the term for a larger-than-normal, increased gap between your two rectus abdominus muscles down the midline of your body.

There is a lot of attention on this lately. There are fitness programs and professionals claiming to rid you of your "mommy tummy" and telling you how bad and dangerous diastasis recti is. It's gotten to the point where I have people asking if they are allowed to do certain activities out of fear because they still have a one-finger gap, and they are wondering if it will cause harm to their body.

A one-finger gap is normal. A two-finger width gap is normal. The abdominal muscles aren't supposed to be touching. There is a small natural separation between the rectus abdominus muscles by the connective tissue called the linea alba. When the spacing is greater than two finger widths, then we might begin to mindfully look into your DRA and consider if the presence of a gap is contributing to symptoms interfering with your quality of life.

> "There is no magic exercise that will close a diastasis. The internet has created a frenzy around diastasis recti. While it has helped increase awareness, there is also a lot of misinformation. The fact is that *there is always a gap*. The rectus abdominals are never fused together, so the word *close* is a bit misleading. The term itself, diastasis recti, is also misleading, as it defines it as a gap when it is a much broader condition. I am not even sure *condition* is the right word here. It is more accurate to describe it as a linea alba insufficiency or impairment. As it stands, the world knows it as diastasis recti. There can be a functional

diastasis and a nonfunctional. If you are nonfunctional (unable to create and maintain tension in the linea alba), it doesn't mean you will be nonfunctional forever. *The key to healing a diastasis* is optimizing the pelvic floor. If the floor isn't working as it should be, then all the diastasis exercises in the world won't do much good. Also, it is not about the exercise. It is about how *you* do an exercise. What is your strategy? Is your strategy taking you towards your goal? Is your strategy helping you manage symptoms and pressure? See a pelvic floor physiotherapist and focus on pelvic floor exercise first, and you will consequently see change in your abdomen and inner core."

—Kim Vopni, The Vagina Coach

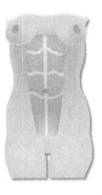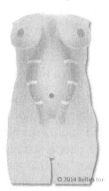

Should you be concerned about this? Your midsection ideally should not bulge/cone/dome out when you're moving because this signals some sort of pressure management imbalance. There are specific ways to make sure you're engaging your pelvic floor and transverse abdominal muscles prior to and through movement to help stabilize and manage your intra-abdominal pressure. There are also ways to monitor your breathing patterns and posture to ensure a better flow of pressure inside your body so that it doesn't bulge forward at the linea alba. There are ways you can eat healthfully to help restore the healing of connective tissue. You can work on massaging tight abdominal muscles that may be causing strain on this separation.

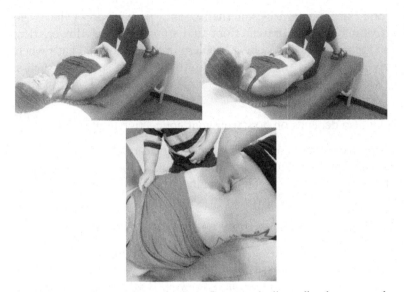

Photos: Check for DRA by putting your fingers at the linea alba above, at, and below the belly button, then lift your head and shoulders up. Check the quality of tension and the number of fingers you can fit between the rectus abdominis. Note any pressure or pain.

When it comes to DRA and function, the main goal is to make sure that you aren't limited in doing your daily activities or fitness routine due to the DRA and that you have no aches or pains at the abdomen, back, hips, pelvis, pubic bone, or anywhere in the body. If DRA is present and you are not properly using your abdominals to support the muscle and fascia connections to the pubic rami, this could present as a complaint of pubic bone pain. You should not be experiencing complaints of leakage or feelings of falling out. The idea is to find strategies that allow you to move without the bulge and feel strong in your connection to muscles in that area. There is a degree of natural separation that occurs while you're pregnant, and if you are planning on having more pregnancies in the future, it's a good idea to attempt to close the gap and make things more functional by learning better movement strategies prior to getting pregnant again or while pregnant still.

There are some online programs that are pretty good at getting you stronger with DRA, but also keep in mind that it's not the specific exercise that's often curing you. It's all about the strategy you're using and how you're applying it with the exercises and real life. Sometimes this gap is a result of over squeezing your upper abs (rectus abdominis and obliques) when doing ab exercises, which can create large pressures internally, and if you don't have good activation of your pelvic floor and transverse abs (lower, deeper abdominals), there may be a problem in this strategy. That's where it may be beneficial to try seeking out a postnatal specialist such as a pelvic floor PT or a fitness instructor specialized in this to get feedback.

A lot also depends on how well your connective tissue heals.

There may be extreme cases where surgical repair may be your best option. But like with most surgeries, try conservative approaches first to really improve your strength and coordination. This will help you immensely in your recovery post-op.

Aesthetic concerns with or without the gap

For the record, I really hate the term mommy tummy, but I know it gets used a lot and that I have many people ask me specifically how to get rid of it. So this section is for you. If you're concerned about a roll at your midline, make sure that first you've learned to properly activate and relax your pelvic floor and transverse ab muscles. Understand how to use this strategy so that you can coordinate it well with your breath and movement. If after applying that strategy to your daily life and exercise routine, you still have a pooch in your midsection that you are unhappy with, it becomes a personal choice about how you want to proceed. How big of a deal is your midsection? Is it simply skin that's stretched and lost its elasticity to bounce back? Is it fat? Was it there before you got pregnant? Will it affect your health and movement? How are your eating habits? Do you have any scar tissue in that area from a cesarean birth?

I believe you should work on function and strategy so that it doesn't interfere down the road, but aesthetics aside, I am not here to tell you to lose your mummy tummy.

How you look and feel with your body is a very personal choice. And I will not succumb to shaming anyone for working their butt off to lose the fat or for being okay or happy with where their body is.

> "You *can* love or embrace your body while wanting it to look or perform differently than it does right now. Both of these things can be true at the same time."

Here's the deal:

1. If you eat nutritious food or work out because you hate your body, even if that helps you reach your goals, it's still not true health.

2. If you think a specific aesthetic or performance goal will change your relationship with your body, it's very likely that you'll be disappointed. How you feel about your body is an inside job.

3. Believing that you can't like your body while wanting to change it means that your feelings about your body are limited to aesthetics or performance. There are so many *other* reasons to like your body and feel grateful for it.

4. Believing that you can't like your body while wanting it to be different means that only "perfect" bodies are worthy of affection. Would we apply this logic to our loved ones?

> "Liking or embracing your body *and* working to change it aren't mutually exclusive."
>
> —Molly Galbraith, CSCS (Girls Gone Strong and Moms Gone Strong)

You grew a human inside you and birthed it into this world! You are amazing.

I do think that regardless, if you're pushing your body to make changes or leaving your body as is to its own natural recovery, you should strive to make peace with where you are today. Making peace doesn't mean you can't still try to change, but you're going to be okay mentally and physically if it doesn't.

Some things you can do to help your midsection and/or DRA are:

- Exercise. Get your body moving in positive ways using the strategy suggested above (coordination of posture, breath, pelvic floor, and movement).

- Consider use of online programs that apply this strategy (links in Resources appendix): Julie Wiebe, Herasphere, Moms Gone Strong.

- Consume quality nutrition. Nourish yourself with real, whole foods (veggies, fats, protein). Avoid overly processed and sugary items.

- Walk daily.

- Drink water.

- Consider collagen-enhancing foods and supplements or bone broth.

- Try kinesio tape or rock tape.

- Consider wrapping: Bellies Inc.

- Seek out professional help with a pelvic floor PT or postnatal fitness specialist.

Recap:

1. Diastasis recti is the separation of abdominal muscles, which may or may not contribute to pain and limitations in your function.

2. Working on closing the gap with strategy and healthy habits can help decrease the chance of your DRA worsening with future pregnancies.

3. Don't fall into the trap of being shamed about a mommy tummy, but if it is important to you or you feel it may be contributing to your function, there are resources out there to help you.

4. When seeing articles on DRA, think critically about what the message is and if it's helpful or harmful to your goals and body image.

CHAPTER 6:
POSTURE CONSIDERATIONS FOR MOM

Whether you're a first-time mom or a sixth-time mom, here are some postures you may encounter specific to taking care of newborns and kids. Like I mentioned in my first book, you should be able to move your body in all different directions. There's no specific bad versus good postures. However, under load and repetition, there may be some ways to optimize your body's muscles and structure. The key is to mix it up. If you've been in the same posture for a long time, move around and switch to a new one.

Try to avoid always doing things one-sided

We know that it's good for a baby's development to change up the side they move and look to. The same applies to us.

As you change your baby's diaper, change the direction in which you put the baby's head so that baby can change the way they're looking at you and that you can mix up the way you use your arms.

Change up the way you cross your legs if you notice that you always sit on your right leg or with your right leg crossed over your left. Try mixing it up. How does it feel to do it with the left leg? How does it feel to sometimes sit symmetrically without crossing? Mix up where and how you sit: on a chair or on the floor in different positions.

Change up the way you lean to your right or left hip in standing. Ideally, try not to lean all the time. See if you can stand with upright posture. If it's difficult or uncomfortable to stand symmetrically for long periods, try to put your foot on a stool to unload the leg instead of jutting the hip to the side.

When carrying bags or a car seat, try mixing up the arm you use. Maybe carry with the left arm into where you're going and use the right arm to carry on your way out.

Try to change up the side you hold the baby on. Mix up the arm you use to feed your baby with or the breast you use.

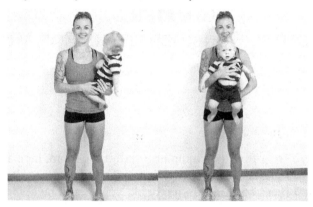

Breastfeeding and bottle feeding

There are a lot of different ways you can hold your baby while feeding. Making sure your baby is comfortable and able to feed is probably top of your radar, but don't forget that you need to also find your most comfortable posture too. This will be a repetitive task, and it's key to make sure you have options to work smarter, not harder. Bring baby to you, not you to baby. This will help you in avoiding too much strain on your neck and shoulders. Use pillows, blankets, or specific breastfeeding pillow like a boppy pillow to prop up the baby to make this possible and sustainable. Feed lying down on your side sometimes.

Mix it up. If you're unsure about your posture, try taking some diaphragm breaths. Do the breaths feel full in all directions: chest, belly, and ribs on the side and in the back all expanding equally? Move forward, back, and side to side until you find a posture that allows you to take nice, symmetrical, full breaths. Using a nursing stool or sitting in a chair that allows you to have your feet supported on the ground can help support the rest of your body.

"I'd recommend referring to a lactation consultant and postpartum doula as well. There are specific ways the baby needs to access the breast to ensure good latch, all while mom is remaining ergonomic."

—Melissa Stendahl, PT, DPT

"Be mindful of your wrist position and keep them neutral to avoid strain. Bring baby to breast, *not* breast to baby. Move your neck slowly while nursing to avoid strain: nod your neck up, down, rotate side to side, and bring your ear to shoulder (no shoulder hiking). Perform gentle neck and upper body stretches after nursing or throughout the day to prevent strain or discomfort in these areas: roll shoulders forward and backward, squeeze your shoulder blades together, perform a genie stretch, and lie on a foam roller parallel to your spine, stretching your arms in a T position. Nursing is a wonderful time to mindfully breath and relax your muscles (especially the pelvic floor) while you bond with your baby. These tips can be applied to bottle-feeding mamas and dads too."

—Dr. Rachel Elizabeth Miller, PT, DPT, IHPS, WHC

Carrying and holding baby

Many options exist for babywearing for different ages and ranges of activities that you're participating in. Look in your area to see if there are any babywearing resources where you might be able to try on different options before making a purchase so that you know what works best for you. Regardless of babywearing or not, you're still going to have to lift and carry your baby. Mix up where and how you're carrying the baby.

Lifting baby, car seats, and other large objects

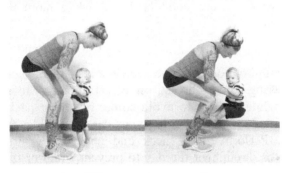

Deadlift   Squat

If you're picking up a baby from ground level, consider a squat or deadlift position to optimize your use of your posterior chain: butt, leg, and back muscles. Keep your baby close to you as you lift. As your baby gets older or if you have toddlers around, encourage them to do most of the work. Ask them to climb up to you if you are sitting in a chair, or if you need to carry them, have them crawl up to something higher so it's easier for you to reach them. Have them help getting in and out of the car so you don't have to do all the work. Although at first it may add a little time and patience, most kids are happy to help, and it will give your body a break from the many times you do need to lift and carry.

Remember your exhale, pick up the bean (contract your pelvic floor muscles), and move.

Use this to your advantage as you build up strength and coordination with lifting your baby and other items. Some car seats, strollers, and Pack 'n Plays are odd shapes and awkward to attempt to hold close to your body for a good lift. Do your best and ask for help if you need it, especially early on as you're still healing.

Recap:

1. Find postures in which you can take nice, full breaths.

2. Avoid always doing things one-sided. Mix it up.

3. Work smarter, not harder with feeding. Use pillows. Bring your baby to you. Breathe!

4. Lift by optimizing your legs, butt, and back. Exhale on exertion and use your pelvic floor.

CHAPTER 7:
OTHER POSTNATAL QUESTIONS ANSWERED

Common versus normal

As you recover in your postpartum healing, continue to monitor for what's common versus normal and reach out if you need help with these issues. There's an extensive chapter titled "Common versus Normal" in my first book. But here's the basic run down: common means it happens frequently and that you're not alone in experiencing these things, but just because something is common does not make it normal, which refers to the healthy, natural state.

So urine leakage (or stool or gas), urinary frequency, urinary urgency, pelvic organ prolapse, pelvic pain, and other areas of pain fall into this discussion. Any amount of leakage (even just a little bit) with coughing, sneezing, laughing, jumping, running, or feeling strong urges is not normal, and there are usually ways for you to improve this. Normal urinary voiding should be every two to four hours. Try not to hold past four hours on a regular basis and try not to go sooner than one to two hours on a regular basis while keeping hydrated properly. Pelvic organ prolapse that is symptomatic may feel like pelvic heaviness or like a tampon is falling out.

You may experience some of these things during pregnancy or postpartum. In the first few weeks as your body heals, these symptoms should resolve. If they have not resolved within a month or two postpartum, consider seeking out help for further assessment. These are not things you need to live with, and if they go untreated, they may lead to bigger, more interfering problems down the line. Talk to your provider about a referral to pelvic floor PT to work on these things.

Breastfeeding and breast health

Know that there are breastfeeding resources out there for you and that if you start to have difficulty breastfeeding, you're not alone, and there is help. Breast milk is optimal for many reasons, but the most important thing is that your baby gets fed and that you feel supported in making these decisions. If you start to experience any pain with feeding or a tender area in your breast, you may be starting to get a clogged milk duct. Also, your baby may not be latched correctly, leading to abnormal pull on the nipple instead of whole areola. This can result in inadequate feeds and in breast pain.

Here are some ideas to help:

- Massage your breast.
- Apply warm compresses before feeding.
- Use hand expression.
- Take a warm shower.
- Be on a regular feeding/pumping schedule.
- Take sunflower lecithin supplements.
- Change up the feeding position of your baby including trying dangle feeding.
- Stay active and hydrated.

Lactation consultations and postpartum doulas can help you through this. You can also see a physical therapist for a heated ultrasound treatment with the goal of breaking up the clogged duct with deep heat sound waves.

Mental health

As mentioned briefly in the beginning, if at any point you have concerns about your mental state of well-being, don't be embarrassed. There are many reasons this could be happening as far as hormones and the changes in your life. This is not your fault. Sleep deprivation is so hard on your body. You are not meant to function without sleep. It is important to establish a support system, ideally before the baby comes. It takes a village to raise a child and to support mom during the postpartum period. Know some good mental health providers in your area or online if you happen to have these concerns. Postpartum depression and anxiety don't just happen right after giving birth. They could also happen during other times when your hormones are changing such as when your period returns or when you stop breastfeeding or if you start birth control.

Here is the link for the Edinburgh Postnatal Depression Scale (EPDS): *https://psychology-tools.com/epds/*. Share the results with your healthcare provider. It is a screening tool that does not diagnose depression.

Connect with nature

"If I may suggest one thing that can begin to start an immediate, impactful shift in your health, it would be going outside and spending time in nature daily or as often as possible. Research on chronic pain and stress both support this simple but powerful practice as an effective means of decreasing pain, reducing stress and anxiety, and increasing feelings of well-being and connectedness with something that is bigger than us. Whether it is thirty minutes on your lunch break, or a remote weekend camping in the woods, committing to time spent in nature will create a positive shift in your health."

-Dr. Jaime Goldman, DPT, RYT, Doula

Your new self

"I'm 10 months postpartum. And I'm beginning to feel more like myself instead of a body that just grows and nurtures a baby. I'm growing but into a new, evolving self. Not only I'm nurturing my boys, but also my own needs, goals, and interests. Early motherhood and pregnancy is a pause. It's temporary, and I am absolutely still in it, but not in the way I was a few months ago, or really, the past one and a half years. The sacrifices evolve, of course. They are always present, just in new ways. Transformation is not about aesthetics — that's one small, insignificant byproduct of postpartum. It's about the evolution in my own womanhood, healing, athleticism, motherhood. It's not finding my way back to what I was, routine was, or life was. That's a sure way of actively seeking disappointment. It's about progressing forward, adapting, owning the changes and settling into a new physical, mental, and emotional homeostasis... until asked to change again, maybe in less dramatic ways? By not rushing this, not hating my body through this, or resenting the sacrifice that pregnancy and postpartum can take/does take in every way has been the best gift I could have ever given to myself during this vulnerable chapter. I am not a patient person. I have high expectations. I am persistent and competitive beyond what's productive sometimes, but intentionally shifting those athlete brain tendencies has been life-changing for myself, body, healing, mental health, athleticism, and motherhood this time around. I hope you consider joining me in this purposeful shift in messaging, mindset, and actions because this wasn't an available, recommended approach after I had Cade. And I want us all to have this permission. I hope we are able to take in the magnitude of how temporary, beautiful, significant, and fragile this time in our life is. Be in it. Because soon you won't be."

—Brianna Battles, MS, CSCS

Recap:

1. Know what's common versus normal and avoid pushing into activities that cause you symptoms of leakage, pelvic heaviness, or pain.

2. If you run into difficulties with breastfeeding, reach out to lactation consultants, postpartum doulas or other professionals, and/or try some at-home remedies.

3. If you have any concerns at all about your mental health, reach out for help and support.

4. Spend time in nature.

5. Be present, patient, and intentional during this temporary, vulnerable, and beautiful time.

> Every woman should
> have access to a
> PELVIC PHYSICAL
> THERAPIST
> after having a
> BABY
>
> **PELVIC GURU™**

FINAL WORDS

Have some grace for yourself.

Women these days are bombarded with the idea you have to do it all, with the aesthetic idea you should get your body back, all while trying to keep a small human alive.

> "Give yourself permission to leave some boxes unchecked. Be brave and try a little more tomorrow or modify the things that didn't go so well today. Be kind to your body and you'll slowly grow into this new normal."
>
> —Kelly Diehl, PT, DPT

Learn to be at peace and find happiness with your new body and life. Strive for strength, function, and health.

Find a balance that will allow you to work on your healing during this time so that you can be the best new version of yourself for you and your family. Use this book so that you can have your best body after baby — not to be confused with having your previous body before your baby.

> "Every woman should have access to a pelvic physical therapist after having a baby. Many women still do not know that having a pelvic physical therapy evaluation after a baby (cesarean or vaginal) can have a major positive impact over a lifetime! This is standard practice in France, and we believe we can do this across the world! [...] This can help with (and prevent worsening of) urinary leakage, fecal and gas leakage, back and hip pain, abdominal separation, and pelvic organ prolapse. [...] It's never too late, even years after baby! Why wouldn't this be a standard?"
>
> —Tracy Sher, MPT, CSCS

I hope this book helps guide and empower you during your healing postpartum. If you feel you would benefit from a more individual approach, a pelvic floor PT can help, among many other professionals specializing in postnatal care. Getting help now if you need it can be a great step in prevention and a long-term investment in your health. There are links to finding a pelvic floor PT near you in the Resources appendix.

You may also opt for online sessions for your postpartum care so that you can begin working on healing from the comfort of your home. I am available for online sessions along with other pelvic floor therapists through the Vagina Whisperer website (*www.thevagwhisperer.com*).

I want you to own where you are right now and feel empowered about gaining back your ability to use your body, mind, and soul fully. I want you to be able to return to exercise, sex, and life pain free.

I'm cheering you on!

xo
Jen

Personal Experience

I wrote this book based on my professional experience prior to experiencing pregnancy and childbirth myself. I got pregnant shortly after I published *Your Best Pregnancy Ever* and *Your Best Body after Baby*. Here I will include my blog posts about my own experiences postpartum. All blog posts were originally published on the Vagina Whisperer website (*https://www.thevagwhisperer.com/*) and can still be found there, including my outdoor home birth story (which is also included in the end of Book 1).

JEN'S POSTPARTUM STORY

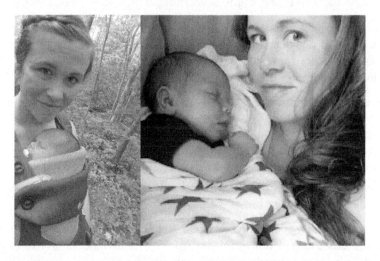

As we wrap up 2019 and head into 2020 I reflect back on the birth of my first daughter and the amazing outdoor home birth I experienced. And I also reflect on the ups and downs of my fourth trimester.

Immediately following the birth of Rowan, I was full of adrenaline, happiness, excitement, accomplishment   and looked forward to bonding. But then it was a blur.

The huge hormonal and identity shift was unlike anything I've ever known. I'm now 6 months postpartum as I write this blog and to be honest the first days and weeks are a bit of a haze. It's hard to know how long certain moments of highs and lows lasted. In hindsight, there's a lot of things I would have chosen to do differently that may have helped me navigate this time. But it is what it is. It challenged me (and my partner), but we grew through it. I learned a lot. And out obstacles comes a whole new appreciation for the things that do go smoothly.

EARLY POSTPARTUM/BABY BLUES/HORMONAL SHIFT/IDENTITY SHIFT

I remember within the first few days postpartum questioning if I would ever feel like myself again. I questioned if I was ready to be a parent. I questioned if I would ever sleep again. I questioned if I would know how to calm my baby. Do I swaddle? Sing? Feed? Pacifier? Change diaper? Is she too hot? Is she too cold? Does she just need to cry? Should I just hold her close and let her cry? Wait this cry feels like she needs something, I just don't know what to give her.

I questioned our decision to have kids. I felt guilt over changing our awesome lives in such a big way. I knew my body needed to rest, but I hated being in my bedroom. I felt claustrophobic in my bed.

As someone who's always been fiercely independent, I didn't want to ask other people to do stuff for me. I knew I could ask others for help if it was needed or to let certain household tasks go, but the problem was that I really felt this urge that I wanted to get up and do them. I wanted to get out and walk the dogs. I wanted to clean up the house or do some laundry. I wanted outer order because I thought it could help keep me calm.

I wanted to sleep, but even when I got the chance I had difficulty getting any sleep. I felt guilty for asking friends and family to hold her to give me a break, so my attempts at rest were usually filled with feelings of shame.

SLEEP WHEN BABY SLEEPS?

I heard several times (and I have often given this advice before my experience), "sleep when baby sleeps", well my baby wasn't sleeping. So here I was: sleep deprived, anxious, baby blues and everyone else seemed to be talking about how their newborns slept all the time. It was hard.

Turns out my baby was hungry. I wasn't producing enough and she was inconsolable. Read more about my breastfeeding and pumping struggles and ultimate decision to switch to formula (next in the 2nd blog post).

The first few weeks were harder than I ever imagined. Yet it could have been so much worse. I realize how lucky I was to have my dream birth experience, be with my health full term baby right away. I was able to be off of work for 9 weeks. I was privileged to even have choices and access to quality care. But there was still a struggle for me in this new role.

Well that covers my huge hormonal shift and feeding struggles. Here's a few other parts of my postpartum story that you may find interesting.

PERINEAL TEARING

I did tear. I had a first degree perineal tear (least severe, perineal skin tear). I chose not to get stitches and let it heal naturally. I looked at the tear with my midwives in making this decision - *that's the pelvic PT in me*. I don't necessarily recommend you do that unless you want to. I did my best to keep my thighs together for the first 7-10 days while things healed. I took short strides while walking, did steps 1 at a time if I needed to, rolled in/out of bed using a log roll with my legs together (and protecting my abs healing). I used SRC compression recovery shorts for support of my perineum and abs. I let the area heal for the first 6 weeks and attempted not to touch it too much. Just some light gentle touch over underwear or gently on skin to decrease my tissue sensitivity but not too much that I was moving any skin. After 6 weeks things had closed completely and I verified tissue healing with my midwives. I then began perineal scar tissue work. You can read more about that in a blog post all about perineal massage.

RETURNING TO EXERCISE

My own experience returning to exercise went pretty smoothly and followed the advice that I often give clients. Take a very individualized approach based on what your body is telling you and what your prior activity level was during pregnancy/pre-pregnancy. The first few weeks I took very small walks increasing daily only a few minutes at a time and increasing the number of walks I did a day. By week 3, I had slowly worked my way back up to a mile walk and by week 4 doing two separate mile walks (one morning, one evening). Around week 6, I started to do a small amount of jog/walk intervals, but it didn't feel super great (pelvic heaviness), so I mostly focused on walking. Already around week 3, I started to slowly add in some gentle pelvic floor exercises with movements: mini squats, mini lunges, bird dogs, fire hydrants, standing hip abduction and hip extension, heel raises, push-ups at a countertop, arm exercises with 8 lb. weights. This was all really scaled back versions of what I was doing during pregnancy. I went to my first crossfit class around 6-7 weeks postpartum and *scaled significantly*. Going at my own pace and number of reps/sets and not keeping track of my totals.

All things I attempted return to within the first 6-12 weeks were things that I regularly did before pregnancy and had continued to be active with throughout my pregnancy. They were also things I could do without pain, leakage, or feelings of falling out/pelvic heaviness. If something didn't feel right I modified. (We can help you with this via our online wellness sessions.)

RETURNING TO SEX

I worked on decreasing my scar tissue sensitivity with touch and massage a few times a week. Once that was feeling better and less painful, I was ready to try some more self-exploration before adding my partner back into the mix. I made sure there was minimal to no pain with pressure along the entire vaginal opening (introitus) and with touch to the deeper pelvic floor muscles inside the vagina. I masturbated to include penetration and with orgasm and was a bit sore after, so I tried this at least one more time before feeling ready to try with my partner. Ready with plenty of water based lubricant, we attempted our first time back at sex post-baby with the communication prior that we're ready to try, but might not go for very long or go to orgasm if it was too much for me. And it went alright. It felt different for me. I could tell I was a bit guarded. I didn't feel like moving much. And I mostly focused on relaxing and breathing. It was slightly uncomfortable around my scar, but overall not painful. Each time after felt a little better, more enjoyable, less guarded, less sore, more ready to move/try various positions again. In the months that followed I still would get a slight twinge near my scar but it was usually decreased with change in position or depth or speed. And as I continued to work on my scar, this was lessening in intensity and frequency.

OTHER THINGS THAT REALLY HELPED ME

- Postpartum perineum and abdomen support: SRC health high waisted compression shorts

- Lots of diapers (for me!) for postpartum bleeding. I found depends easier to use than pads

- Easy to eat/digest foods: Smoothies, bone broths and protein shakes

- Plenty of snacks on hand: nuts, lara bars, fresh veggies/fruits

- Keeping my water glass full!

- Fresh air

- Showering in the morning before my husband left for work. This helped me start my day feeling clean and like I accomplished something.

- "Happy nipples," a locally made nipple balm by Erica Macrum (I have also heard good things about Motherlove and Earthmama organics).

- Having a supportive team including medical (my midwives) and friends/family (food dropped off, baby cuddles, hugs, listening ears, etc.).

- Having a go with the flow attitude. After getting over my initial baby blues and feeding issues, having a calm "we'll just see what happens" attitude really helped ease future decisions for us.

- My partner. A big shout out to my amazing husband, Alex, I don't know how I could have done this without you.

WHAT I WOULD HAVE DONE DIFFERENTLY

- Asked my husband to take 2 weeks of paternity leave. Summers are his busiest season with work so we hesitated to have him take more than 4 days off, but he's my rock and I was really shook without him. I wish I would have had 2 weeks of just us to adjust to this transition.

- Had a formula picked out just in case and/or a source of donor milk, so that I didn't feel so pressured to provide all the food via breastfeeding or pumping (in case there was difficulty with production on my end).

- Once I realized I wasn't supplying enough milk to my baby on my own, I wish I would have surrendered sooner to the idea that I may not be able to *exclusively* provide her food and used a combination of donor milk and/or formula, so that I could try a more relaxed breastfeeding/pumping schedule.

- REST MORE in week 1 and 2. I wish I would have practiced what I preach to clients here. If my husband had been home and our baby better fed, I would hope to create a better set up that felt open/calm to heal and rest in. I spent a lot of time visualizing my birth space. I wish I would have spent more time visualizing my postpartum recovery space.

Here we are six months postpartum. Things are pretty great. We have a very happy, healthy baby. She's so easy going and fun to be with. Her giggles and cuddles are some of my favorite things to look forward to each day.

Just like there's a wide range of birth experiences possible, there can be a variety of postpartum journeys. Some things may be within your control and other things out of your control. Know that you're not alone in this rollercoaster. And if you need further professional help, we're here for you. All of us at the Vagina Whisperer have our own stories to tell, but we're also here to listen to yours. We're here to help you through your postpartum experience.

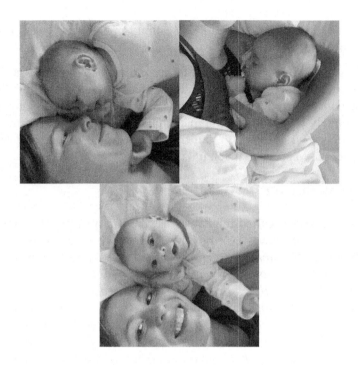

DIFFICULTY FEEDING MY BABY: A STORY OF BREASTFEEDING, PUMPING & FORMULA TRANSITION

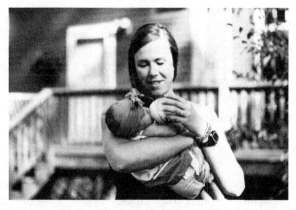

The first weeks postpartum my baby was inconsolable. And something didn't feel right. I didn't know if I was bad at parenting, bad at breastfeeding, or bad at reading my baby's cues. I felt overwhelmed. Turns out my baby wasn't getting enough food.

Luckily, I was able to reach out to my midwives regularly via text, phone calls and home visits. I expressed my concerns and they listened and offered advice. Early intervention led us to realizing that I most likely wasn't producing much milk yet. It's normal for milk to take a few days to come in, but this was different - I may not have the potential to produce much milk.

TUBULAR BREAST DEFORMITY

I have something called tubular breast deformity. Even working in healthcare, I had never heard of this diagnosis before. According to Healthline.com: *Tubular breasts is the name of a condition caused by breast tissue not proliferating properly during puberty. The condition is also called tuberous breasts or breast hypoplasia. While not extremely common, tubular breasts cannot be considered rare because many women don't seek treatment. Tubular breasts are diagnosed based on the way that the breasts look. Researchers are still learning about tubular breasts, so it's a somewhat subjective diagnosis that can take several forms.*

What really helped me was finding this Huffington Post article The condition that stopped me from Breastfeeding. I found this quote comforting that I wasn't alone: "I surrendered the vision of myself as a breastfeeding mother, and began to formula-feed." -Lisa Selin Davis

My baby was latching well and it wasn't that I wasn't producing anything, but it wasn't enough to fill her up. She was sucking so much it was burning a lot of calories while not getting enough in her. I was lucky enough to have a friend willing to share a week's worth of breast milk with me so that I could keep giving Rowan breast milk while I navigated this new obstacle.

TRIAL PUMPING

I started trial pumping while still breastfeeding some. Then I tried exclusive pumping around the clock, every 2 hours including overnight to stimulate production. I slept in a different room the first night I tried this and set alarms every 2 hours: wake up, pump, attempt to syringe out any teeny tiny bit of milk to save for Rowan, rinse the pump and charge it, then back to bed, only to wake up roughly an hour later and repeat. Rowan was being bottle fed the donor milk from my husband during the night.

After just 2 nights of this, it didn't feel right to me. It was hard. I wasn't sleeping and you need sleep and relaxation to produce well. I wanted to be near my baby and my husband. So I loosened up on the pumping regularity and decided just to pump when Rowan woke up to eat. I would pump and my husband would feed her.

But this strategy was also really hard on us. Both of us waking up at the same time. Losing precious sleep that we could be trading off or be more relaxed during. I was also trying various foods, drinks, teas and other herbal remedies. Which all costs money.

IS IT THE PUMP?

Then I started to question my actual pump. I chose to use the Elvie pump which is a hands-free mobile pump, buttttt you're not able to see if/how much you're pumping in real time (the pump is concealed inside your bra) and I wouldn't know until the end of the session if I got anything out at all (it's supposed to tell you on your phone app how much you're producing but mine was not always accurate at such small amounts).

My midwives were able to lend me a hospital grade pump and for better or worse my results were about the same. I tried to up my frequency of pumping once more, but mentally I was shot. I was taking care of Rowan all day by myself (my husband went back to work on day 4) and it was hard enough to attempt to pump with a hands free pump while caring for/feeding/holding Rowan. She didn't sleep much at all during the day at this point and it was near impossible to care for her while pumping hooked up to a wall.

USING DONOR BREAST MILK

When the first week of donor breast milk was out, an amazing anonymous mama donated a bunch of breast milk to my midwives who in turn shared that with me/Rowan. This was such a relief because during this time I was still really stuck on staying with breastmilk as long as possible (all the breastfeeding books brainwashed me to not try formula yet), but also during this time Rowan started to have gas/upset stomach issues. Her cry was intense and painful to hear and I wasn't sure if it could possibly be a reaction to something in the diet of the breast milk donor mother. Many friends have shared their kiddos had difficulty with digesting certain foods through breast milk such as dairy, broccoli, spicy foods, etc. So I had some difficult decisions to consider going forward.

SWITCHING TO FORMULA

I ultimately hit a point where I was ready to switch to formula as her main source of food. I was ready to let go of the uncertainty of donor milk. I was ready to let go of breastfeeding. And I was ready to let go of pumping. I don't feel like I gave up. I feel like I gave it a decent try and in the end it's not what was going to work best for the happiness and health of our family.

After attempting to exclusively pump for more than a week, there was a moment when Rowan was fussy and I attempted to calm her with breastfeeding. It didn't go as smoothly as it had previously and I knew in that moment it was my last time breastfeeding her. Something I had looked forward to doing to provide for her was over. But at the same time, I felt at peace with my switch to formula and a huge weight was lifted. I mean huge. I calmness came over all of us. Our entire family.

MAKING PEACE

I feel so privileged I was able to take the time to research a formula I was content with. I chose HiPP (dutch version). I'm grateful I have the financial resources to provide such a high quality formula to my baby. I'm grateful to the donor milk she was able to eat while we worked on making this decision and exhausting milk production possibilities. I'm grateful we were able to experience some breastfeeding.

In total I probably only breastfed up until week 2-3 and pumped until week 4. I'm not sure on exact dates because I was in quite a fog. But when we made the switch to a consistent formula, wow. Baby was fed. Baby started sleeping better. I felt I could parent better. I could use all the time I was devoting to pumping to being there for my baby, myself and my partner. I was sleeping. I could breathe again.

I'm so in awe of the mamas who commit to breastfeeding and pumping, who work through struggles of latching, overproduction and underproduction. Who find ways to fit this in to provide for their baby. But I also have a whole new respect for mamas who know this road is not for them, whether by choice or not.

I had a friend who shared with me during this time that she hated breastfeeding and instead exclusively pumped. I had another friend who shared with me that she couldn't stand pumping or breastfeeding and hated every minute of it. This honesty helped me cope. Yes, breastfeeding has many amazing benefits. Our bodies are magical. But, it is important that your baby does get fed and that you feel healthy as well. Whatever decision feels right for you, explore it and own it. I read multiple breastfeeding books prior to birth, but I did not prepare for what formula I might want to use to supplement or switch to if things didn't work out. As a planner, that is something I wish I would have taken the time to do. I wish I would have felt okay with using formula to supplement earlier while still attempting to breastfeed a small amount as this may have put less pressure on me.

Being able to feed my baby was a rollercoaster of emotions. I put so much pressure on myself. And I had a lot of healing to do about not being able to supply her with my own milk. I had a lot of healing to do in loving my body. There's so many reasons why someone may choose (or not have a choice) in the way they feed their baby. Let's support one another in all our journeys.

YOUR BEST BODY AFTER BABY CHECKLIST

To keep track of some of the healthy habits for healing in your fourth trimester, I created Your Best Body after Baby checklist to help you reach your goals. Every woman will heal differently and should approach this time (and checklist) in your own way. Listen to your body and go at a pace that feels right to you. This is YOUR journey, be in it and give yourself grace. Here are just some ideas. You got this! Xo Jen

WEEK 1	Day 1	2	3	4	5	6	7
Drink water							
Eat nutritious foods							
Pain relief for perineum							
Have a bowel movement							
Sleep when you can							
Start diaphragm breathing							
Take small walks (less than 5 min at a time) to promote circulation							

WEEK 2	Day 8	9	10	11	12	13	14
Drink water							
Eat nutritious foods							
Sleep when you can							
Add gentle pelvic floor exercises to breathing							
Exhale with exertion (sit to stand, lifting, bending)							
Take small walks (less than 10 min)							

DID YOU ENJOY THIS BOOK?

It would be really awesome if you would leave a review on Amazon so others can find out if this book would be helpful to them.

I truly appreciate you taking the time to do that.

ACKNOWLEDGEMENTS

Using my platform to empower women would not be possible if it weren't for

- The contributions of those that paved the way: Julie Wiebe, Tracy Sher, Brianna Battles, Marika Hart, Sara Reardon, Shelly Prosko, Amy Stein, and many more!

- The mentorship of Meagan Peeters-Gebler.

- The support of Orthopedic & Spine Therapy.

- The UW-La Crosse PT program and especially my partner in all things pelvic, Kelly Diehl.

- All of my wonderful clients I've had the pleasure of working with.

- All the support of my family and friends!

RESOURCES

Find a PT near you:

- Pelvic Guru: Find a Pelvic Health Professional: https://pelvicguru.com/2016/02/13/find-a-pelvic-health-professional/

- American Physical Therapy Association Section on Women's Health PT locator: http://pt.womenshealthapta.org/

- Herman & Wallace | Pelvic Rehabilitation Institute: https://pelvicrehab.com/

Links to those providing quotes and support:

Introduction

- Brianna Battles, MS, CSCS

  o Everyday Battles: Strength and Conditioning: www.briannabattles.com

- Dr. Jaime Goldman, DPT, RYT, Doula

  o Luna Physical Therapy: www.lunaphysicaltherapy.com

Chapter 1: Rest and Healing

- Marika Hart, APA-Titled Musculoskeletal Physiotherapist, BSc (Physiotherapy), MSc (Manual Therapy)

  o Founder of Herasphere: https://herasphere.net

  Full blog post: https://herasphere.net/pelvicfloor/need-know-early-days-post-c-section/

- Meagan Peeters-Gebler, PT, DPT, CMTPT, CSCS

  o Orthopedic & Spine Therapy, Appleton, WI http://www.ostpt.com/therapists/meagan-peeters-gebler/

- Kelly Diehl, PT, DPT

o Vernon Memorial Healthcare

- Chelsea Fanchi, birth doula

  o Chequamegon Doulas:
  https://www.chequamegondoulas.com/

- Sara Reardon, PT, DPT, WCS, BCB-PMD

  o The Vagina Whisperer: https://www.thevagwhisperer.com/

  o NOLA Pelvic Health:
  https://www.thevagwhisperer.com/nola-pelvic-health-physical-therapy/

Chapter 2: Returning to Exercise

- Sara Reardon, PT, DPT, WCS, BCB-PMD

  o The Vagina Whisperer: https://www.thevagwhisperer.com/

  o NOLA Pelvic Health:
  https://www.thevagwhisperer.com/nola-pelvic-health-physical-therapy/

- Julie Wiebe, PT

  o Julie Wiebe PT www.juliewiebept.com

  o Online courses:
  http://www.juliewiebept.com/products/online-courses/

- The diaphragm pelvic floor piston demo:
  https://www.youtube.com/watch?v=mLFfZfm7O7c

- The diaphragm and the internal pressure system:
  https://www.youtube.com/watch?v=cW9mwfy-6-I

- Pelvic floor model

  o Pelvic Model: http://esp-models.co.uk/composite-pelvispelvic-floor

- Kelly Diehl, PT, DPT

  o Vernon Memorial Healthcare

- Haley Shevener, CSCS

  o Pre/postnatal Fitness with Haley Shevener:
  https://www.haleyshevener.com/

o Full blog post:
https://www.girlsgonestrong.com/blog/female-fitness/why-
playground-workouts-can-be-a-parents-best-fitness-friend/

Chapter 3: Returning to Sex

- Sara Reardon, PT, DPT, WCS, BCB-PMD

    o The Vagina Whisperer: https://www.thevagwhisperer.com/

    o NOLA Pelvic Health:
    https://www.thevagwhisperer.com/nola-pelvic-health-
    physical-therapy/

Chapter 4: Optimizing Scar Tissue

- Abigail Inman, PT, DPT

    o Aurora West Allis Medical Center

    o Full blog post:
    https://www.fromabbywithlove.com/blog/2018/6/26/cesarean-
    recovery

Chapter 5: Let's Talk Diastasis Recti

- Kim Vopni, the Vagina Coach

    o Founder of Pelvienne Wellness Inc:
    www.vaginacoach.com

    o Cofounder of Bellies Inc: www.belliesinc.com

- Molly Galbraith, CSCS

    o Cofounder and owner of Girls Gone Strong:
    https://www.girlsgonestrong.com/

    o Cofounder and owner of Moms Gone Strong:
    https://go.girlsgonestrong.com/quiz-page

    o Creator of the Coaching & Training Women Academy:
    https://academy.girlsgonestrong.com/

- Programs mentioned:

    o Julie Wiebe: http://www.juliewiebept.com/products/online-
    courses/#Individuals

    o Herasphere: https://herasphere.net/postnatal-online-
    program/

- o Moms Gone Strong: https://go.girlsgonestrong.com/quiz-page

- o Bellies Inc: https://www.belliesinc.com/

Chapter 6: Posture Considerations for Mom

- ● Melissa Stendahl, PT, DPT

  - o Stendahl PT: https://www.stendahlpt.com/

- ● Dr. Rachael Elizabeth Miller PT, DPT, IHPS, WHC

  - o Physical therapist and women's health coach: http://drrachaelelizabeth.com/

Chapter 7: Other Questions Answered

- ● Dr. Jaime Goldman, DPT, RYT, Doula

  - o Luna Physical Therapy: www.lunaphysicaltherapy.com

- ● Brianna Battles, MS, CSCS

  - o Everyday Battles: Strength and Conditioning: www.briannabattles.com

Final Words

- ● Kelly Diehl, PT, DPT

  - o Vernon Memorial Hospital

- ● Tracy Sher, MPT, CSCS

  - o Pelvic Guru: www.pelvicguru.com

  - o Sher Pelvic Health: www.sherpelvic.com

ABOUT THE AUTHOR

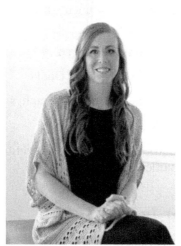

Photo credit: Kelsey Lindsey

My name is Jen Torborg. I'm a licensed physical therapist with a passion for pelvic floor physical therapy. My goal is to empower you on your journey to understanding your body and mind better during pregnancy and postpartum and while dealing with pelvic, bladder, bowel, and sexual dysfunction. I am the author of three books in the Pelvic Floor Physical Therapy Series: *Your Best Pregnancy Ever*, *Your Best Body after Baby*, and *Your Pelvic Health Book*.

I received my doctorate of physical therapy (DPT) from University of Wisconsin-La Crosse. I have my Certificate of Achievement in Pelvic Health Physical Therapy (CAPP-Pelvic) and Certificate of Achievement in Pregnancy/Postpartum Physical Therapy (CAPP-OB) from the American Physical Therapy Association (APTA) Section on Women's Health (SoWH). I often incorporate dry needling in my practice, and I am a certified myofascial trigger point therapist (CMTPT) through Myopain Seminars.

I strive to provide a positive, comfortable environment to treat clients in Ashland, Wisconsin at St. Luke's Chequamegon Clinic. I also work with clients virtually through pelvic wellness sessions at The Vagina Whisperer. I look forward to educating my patients about their body and how they can take control of their health.

Outside of my career, I have a love for the woods and the water. I live in the Chequamegon Bay region of Lake Superior. Home is being surrounded by trees and trails with the love of my life, Alex, our daughter, Rowan, and our two dogs, George and Lucy. I enjoy being in nature, which gives me a sense of calm and restores me. I love minimizing and tidying. And I'm inspired by a beautiful sunrise.

Made in the USA
Middletown, DE
21 February 2022